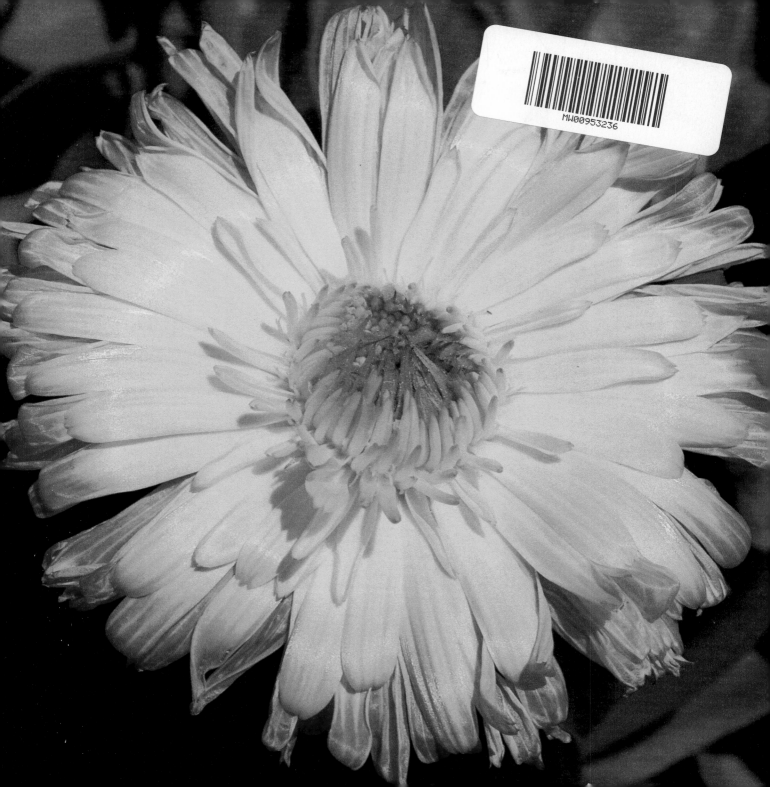

MW00953236

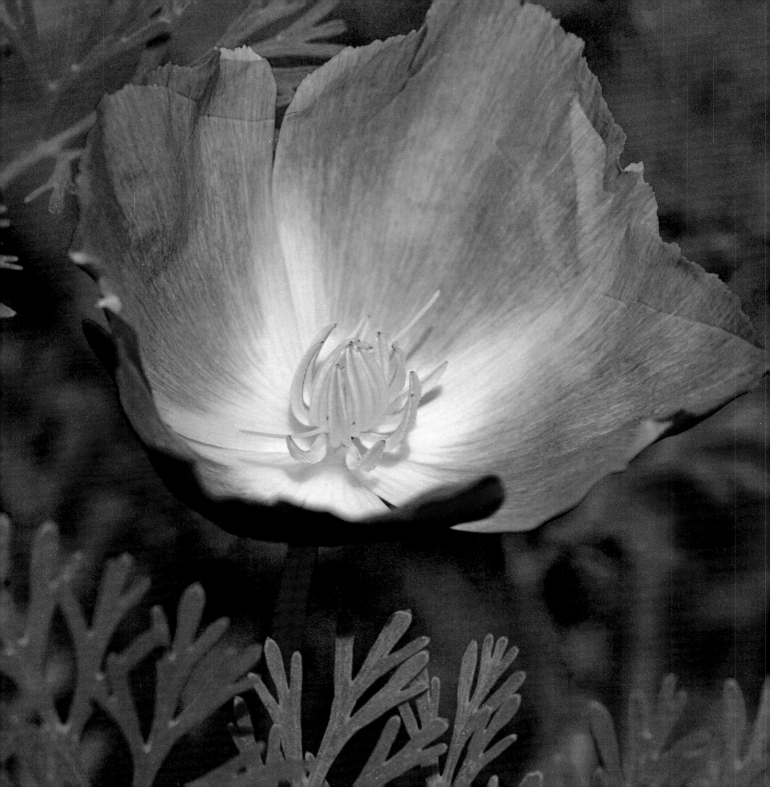

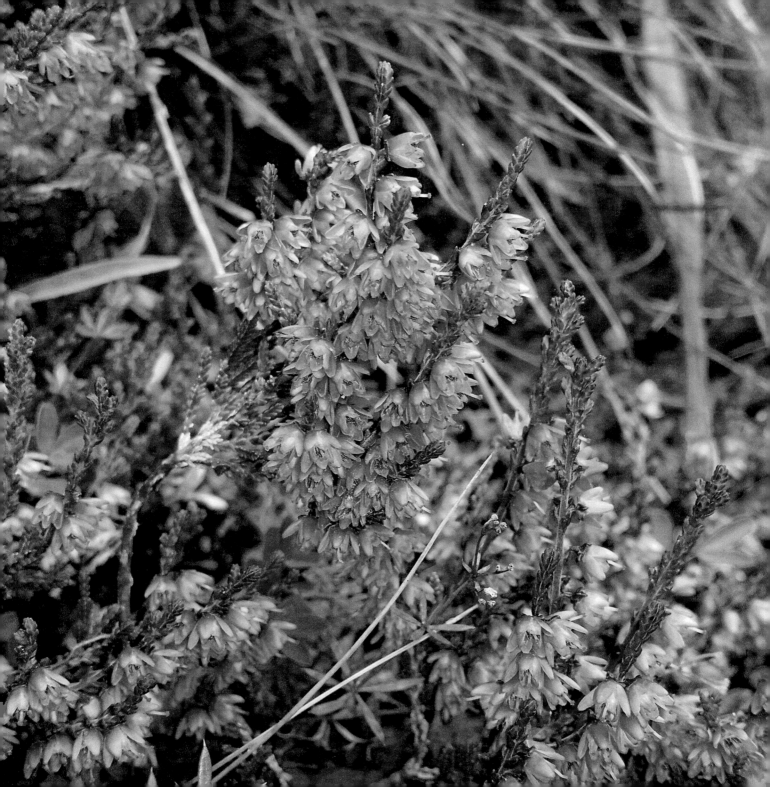

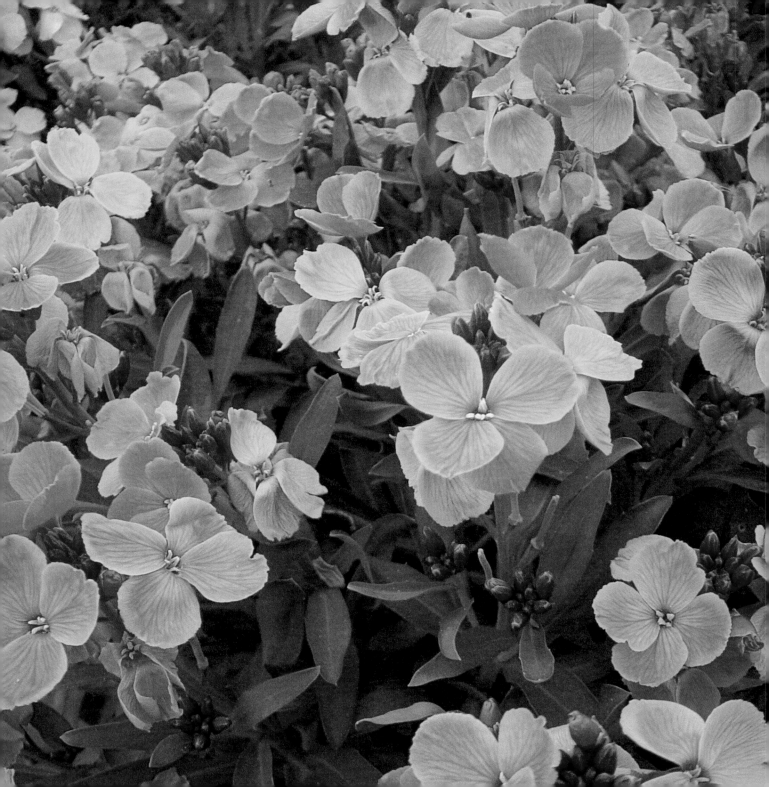

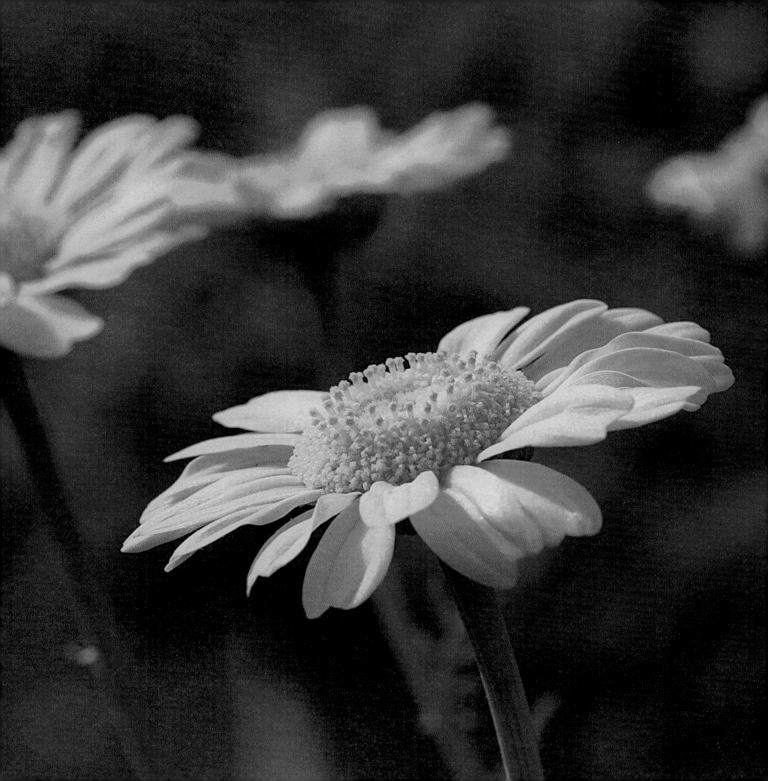

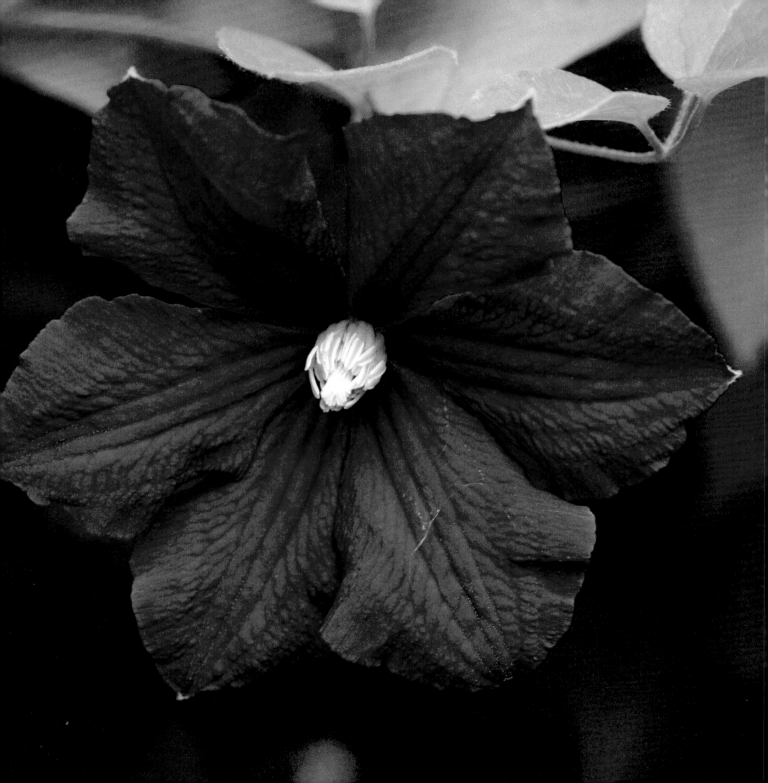

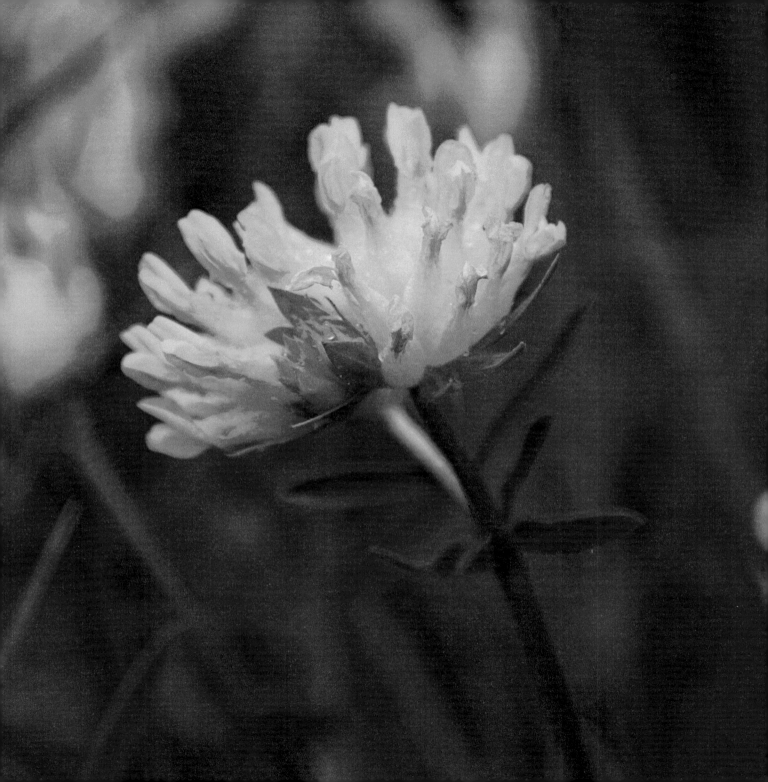

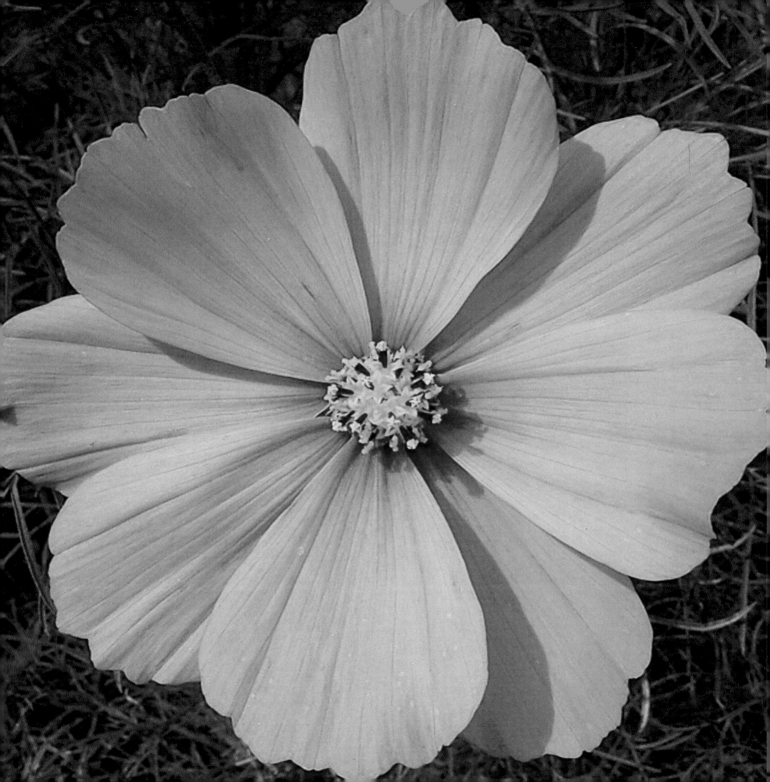

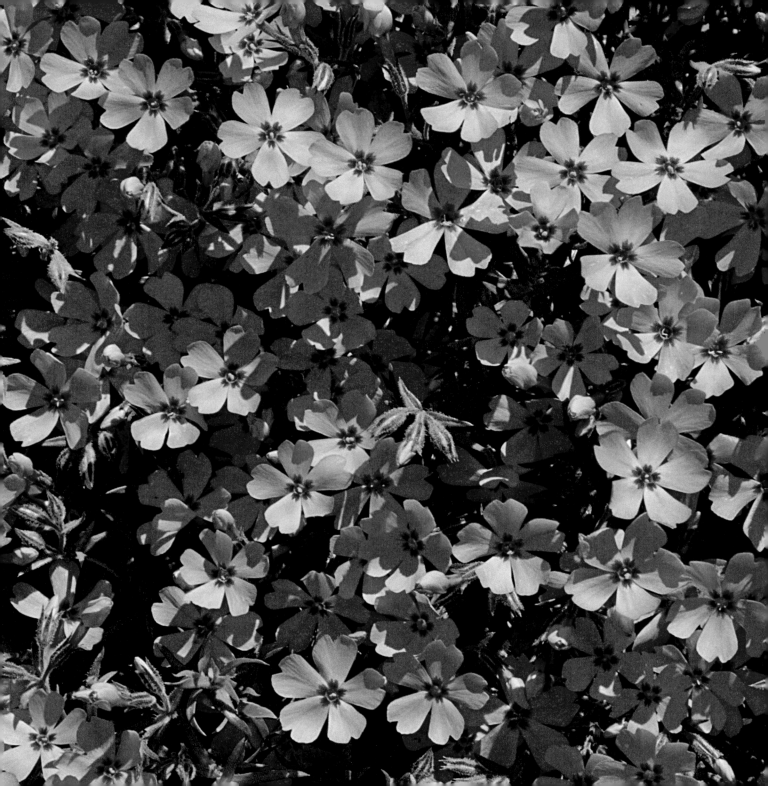

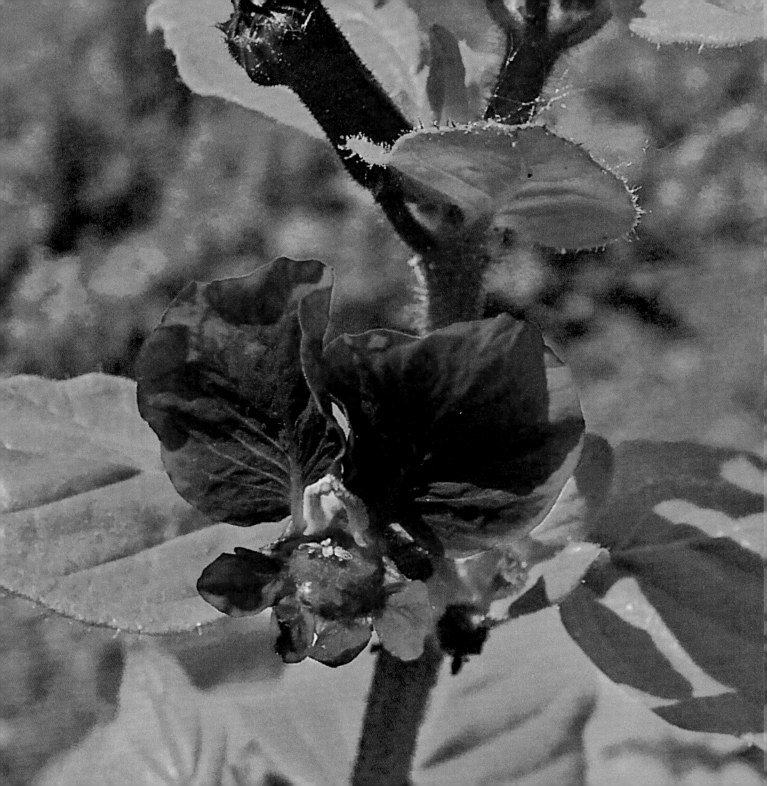

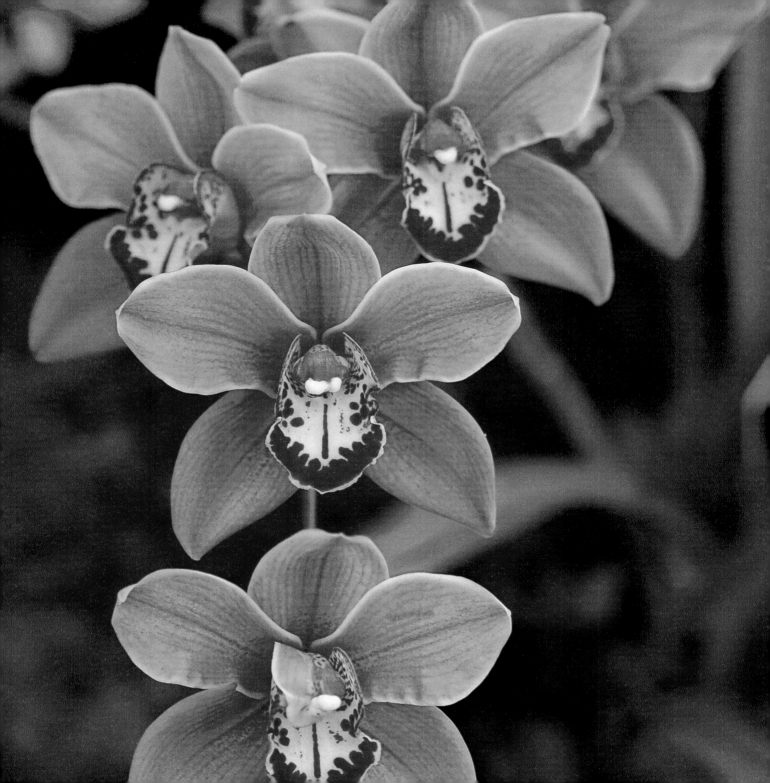

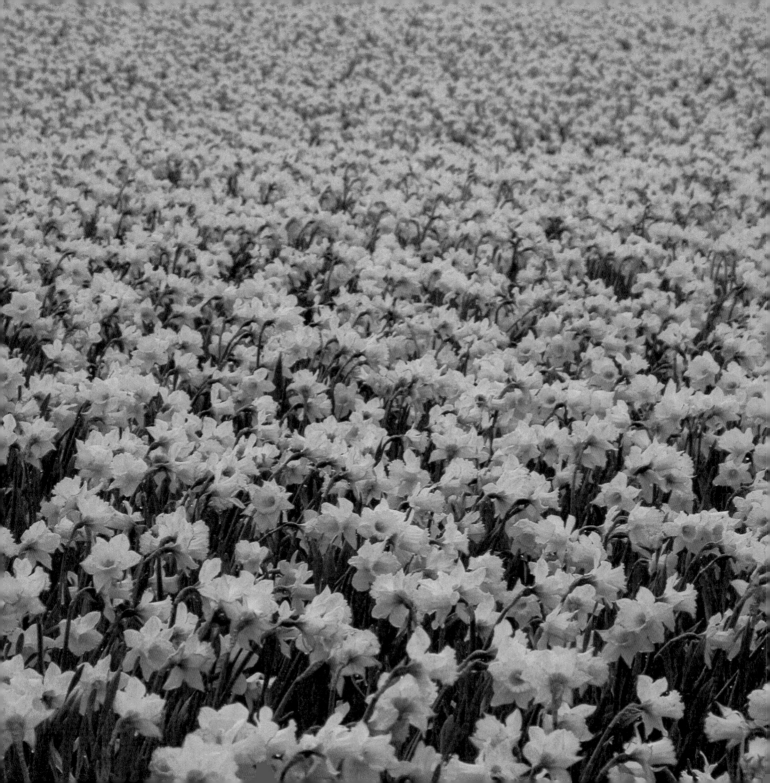

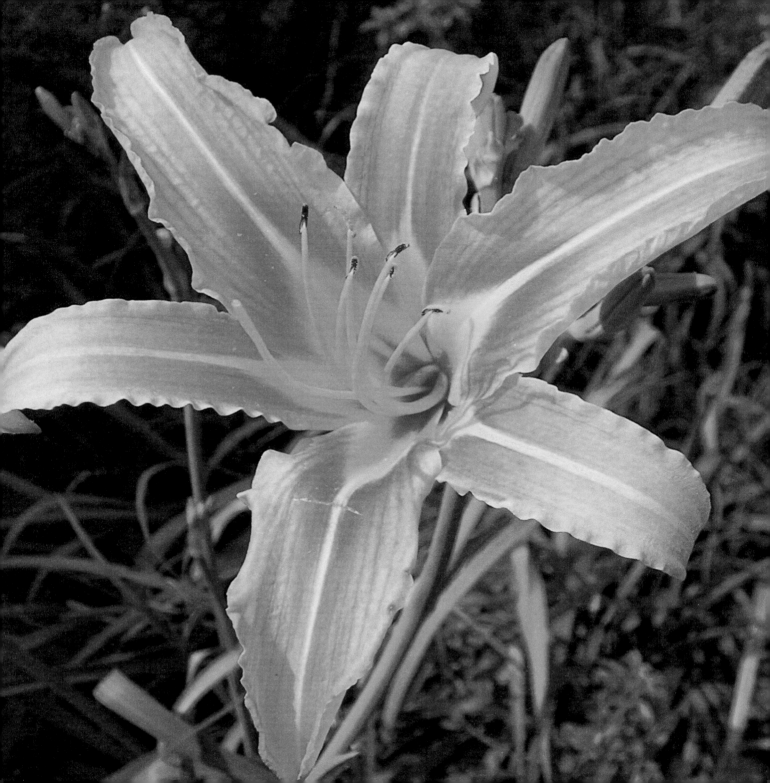

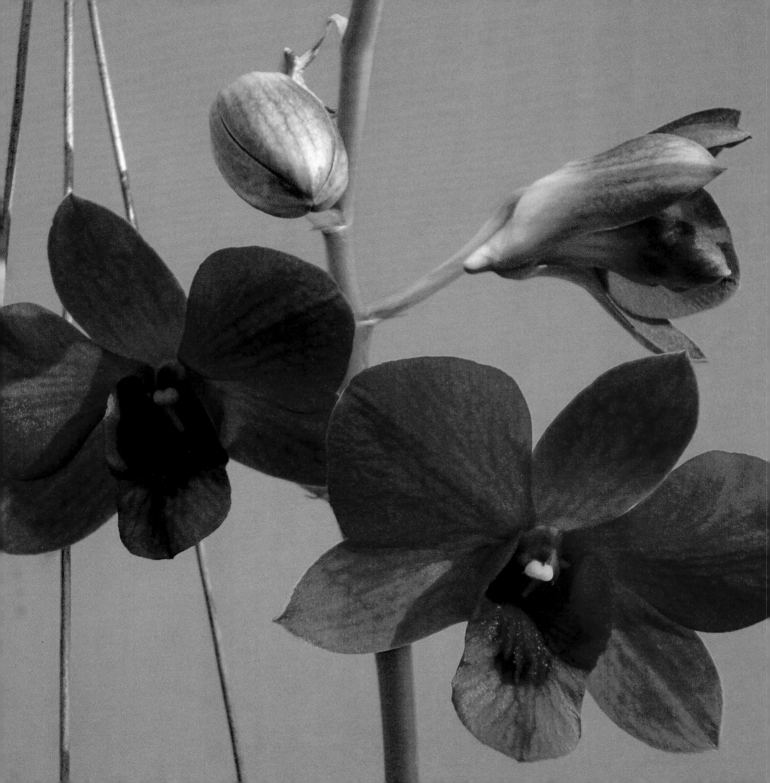

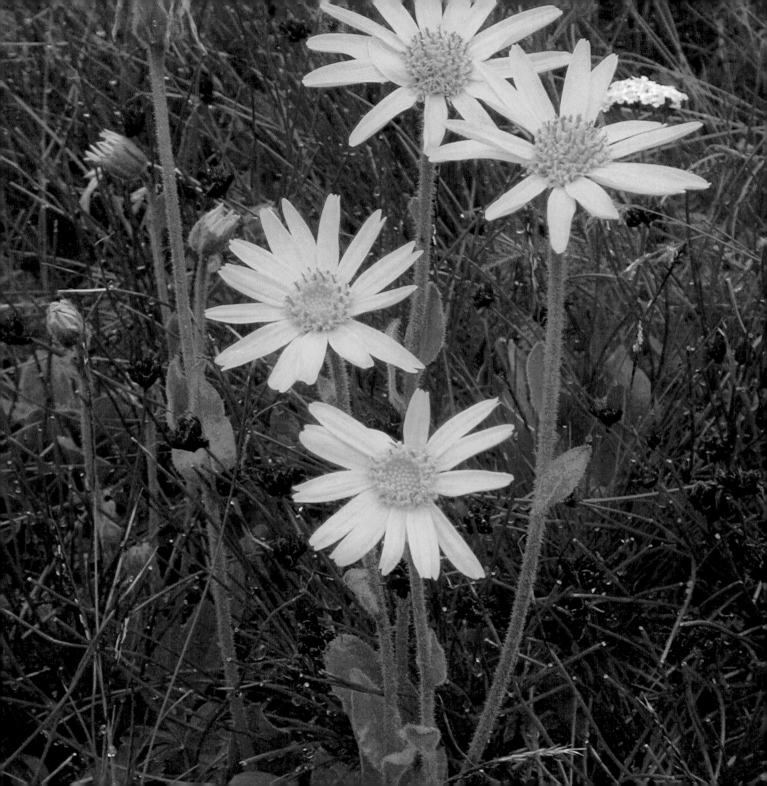

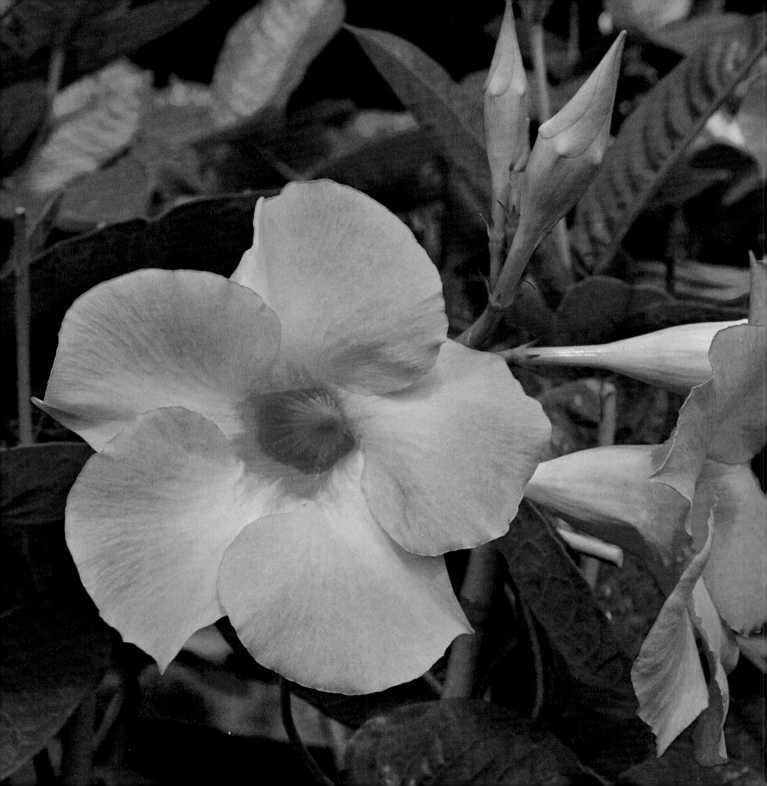

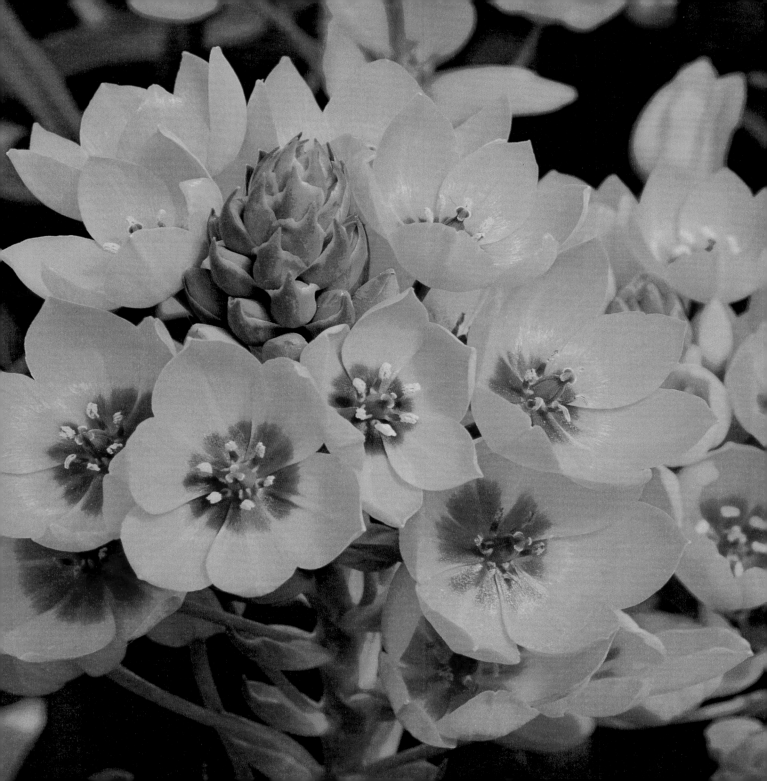

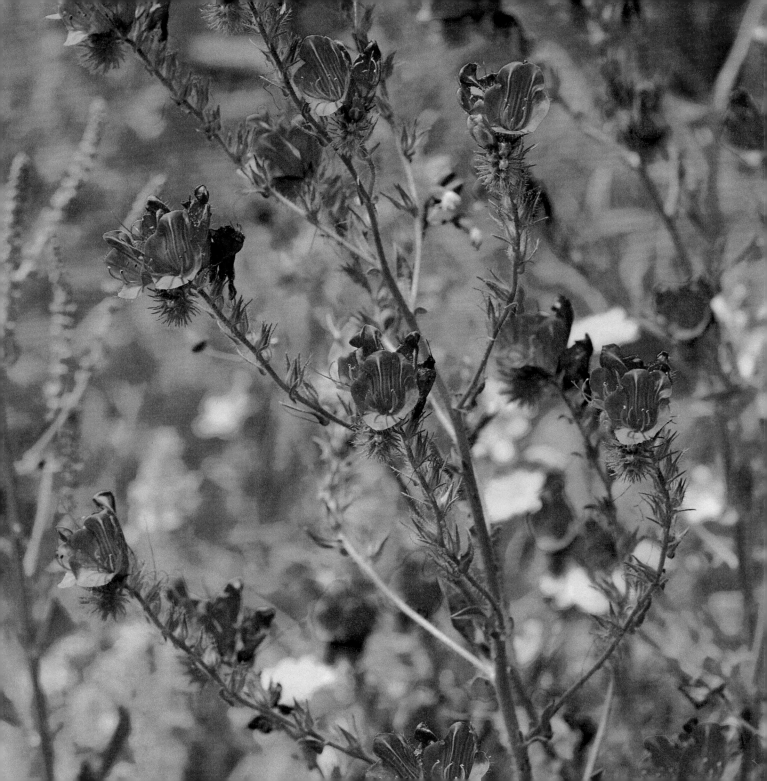

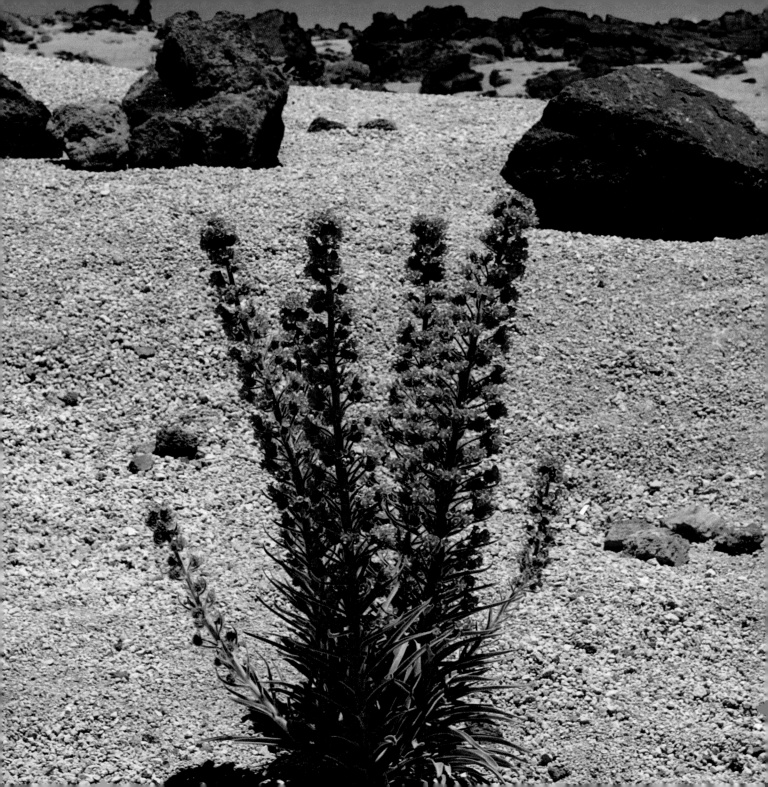

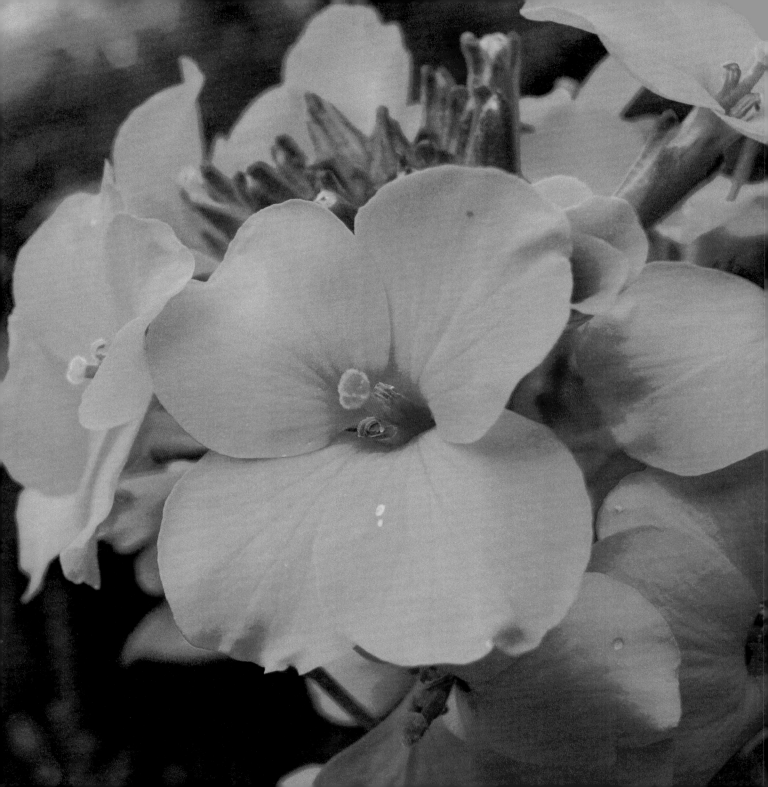

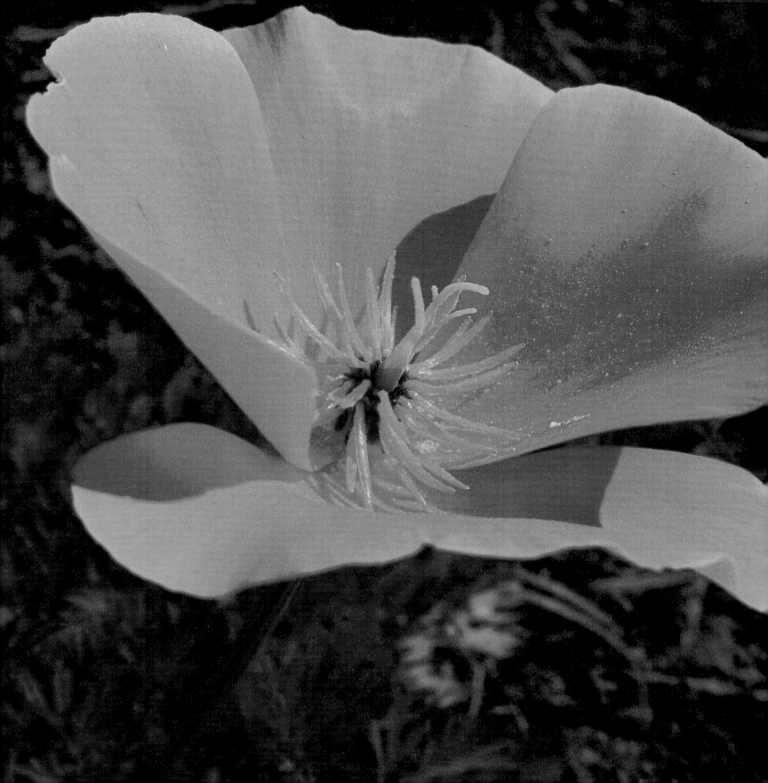

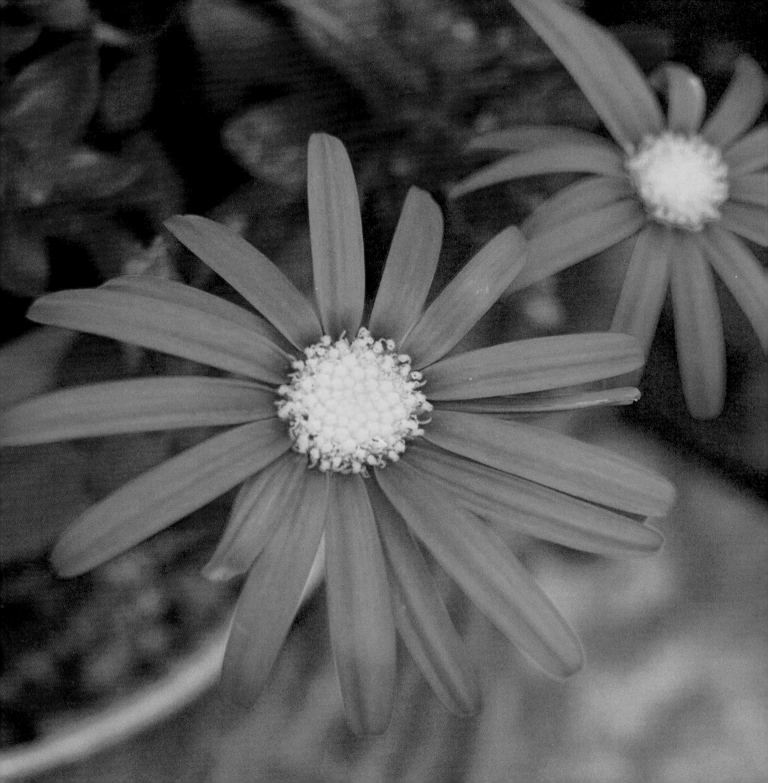

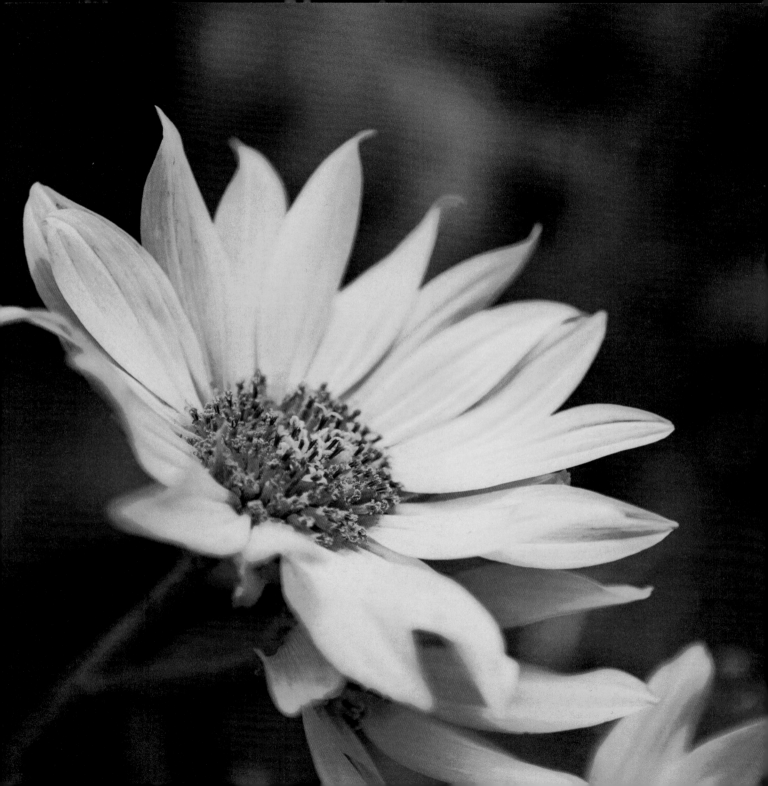

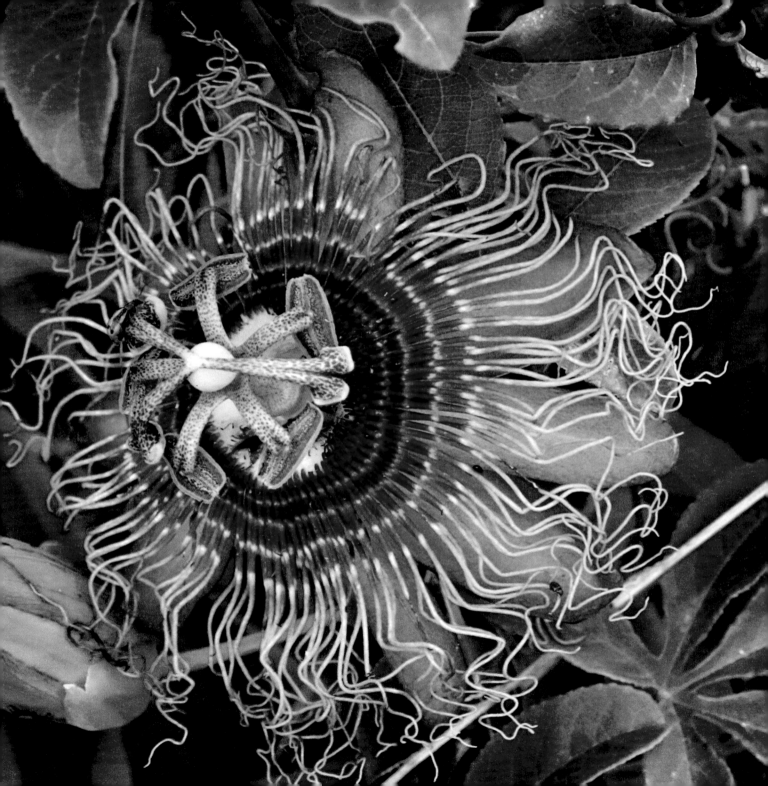

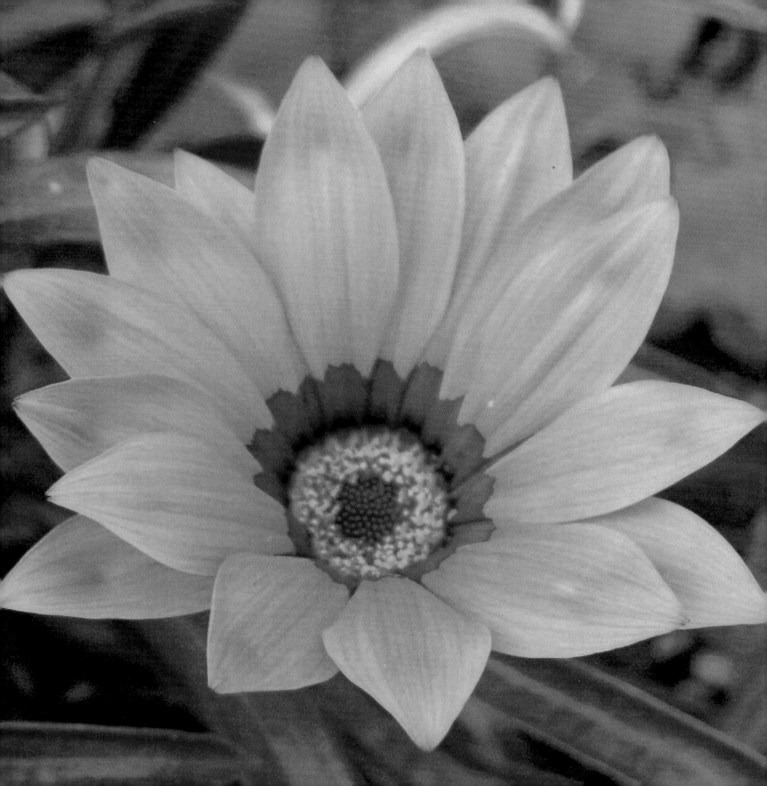

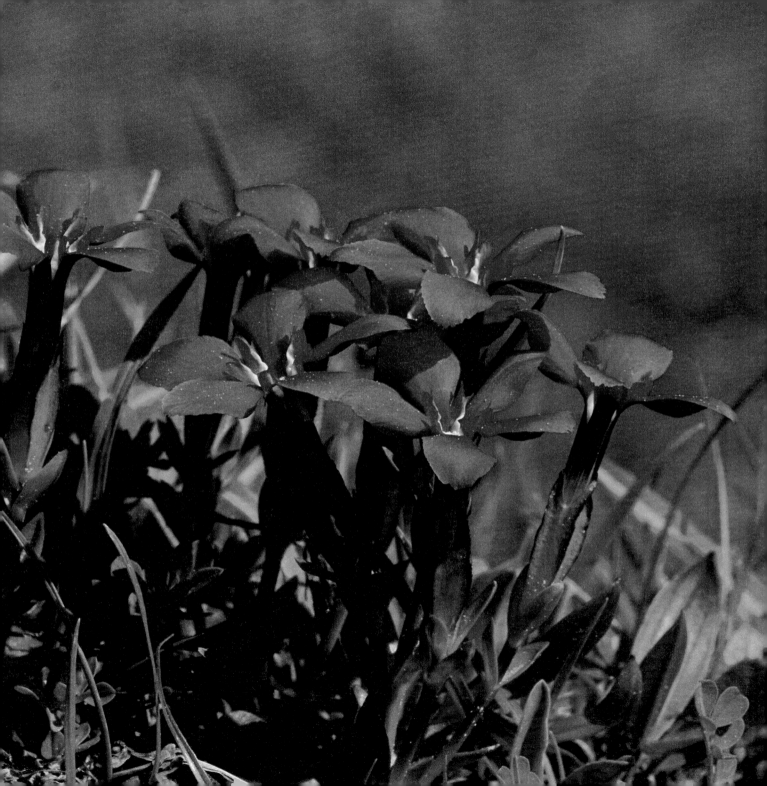

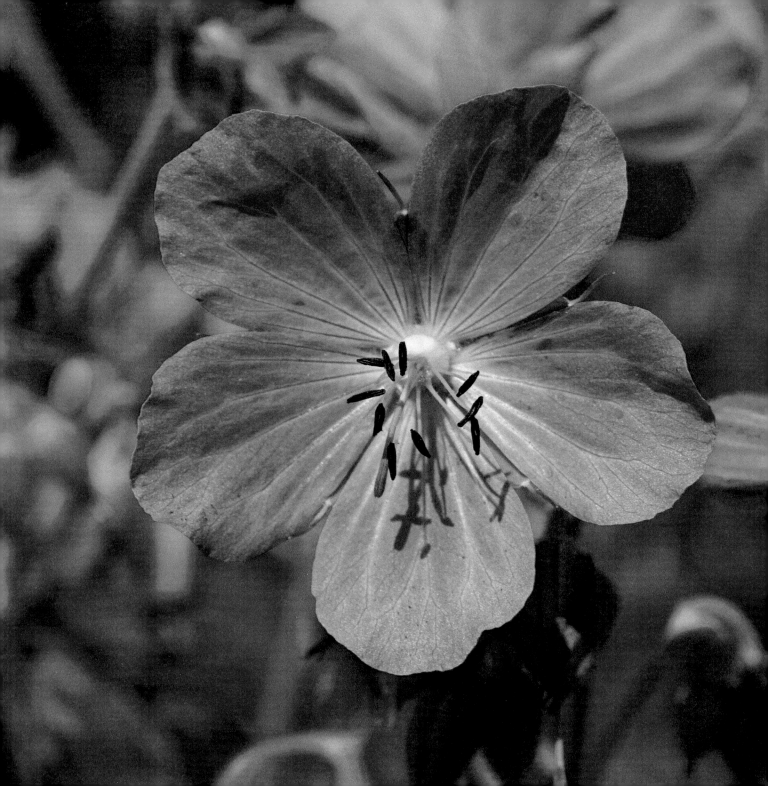

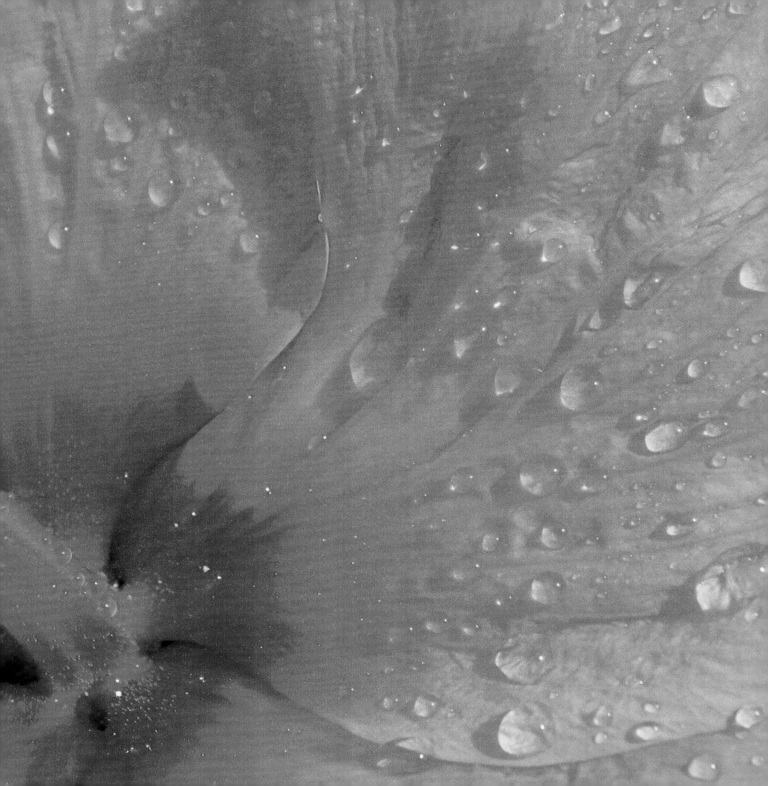

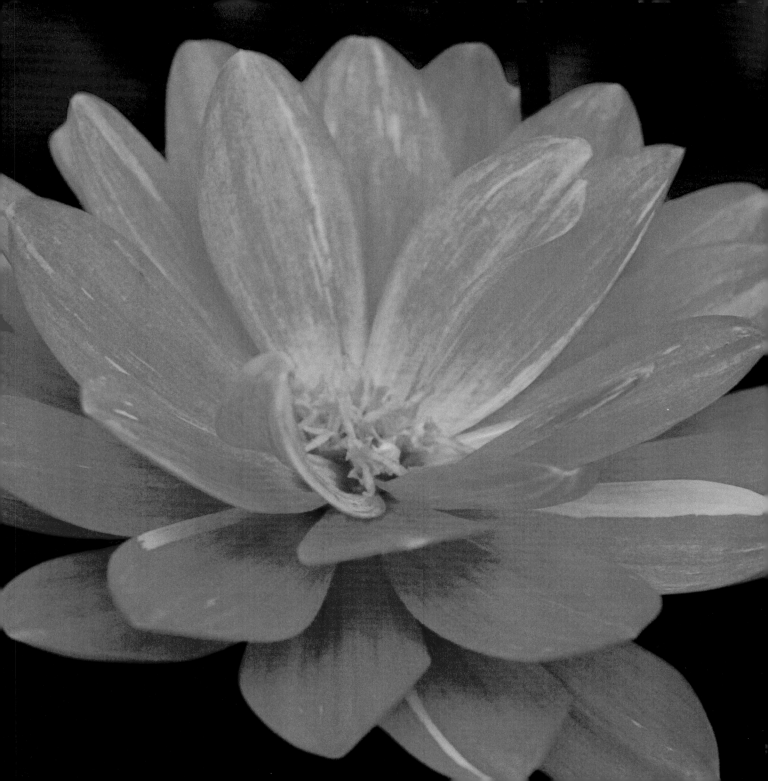

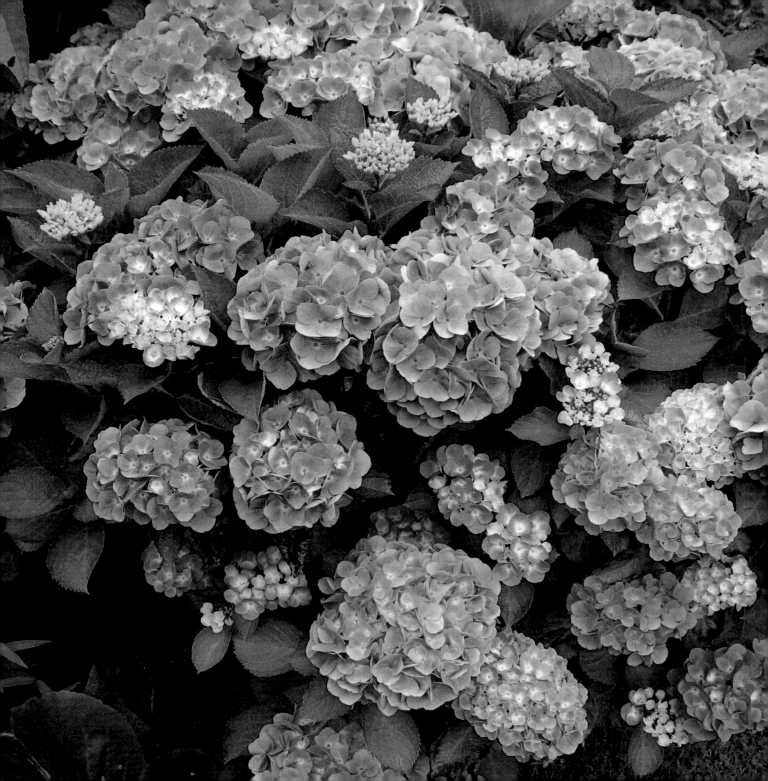

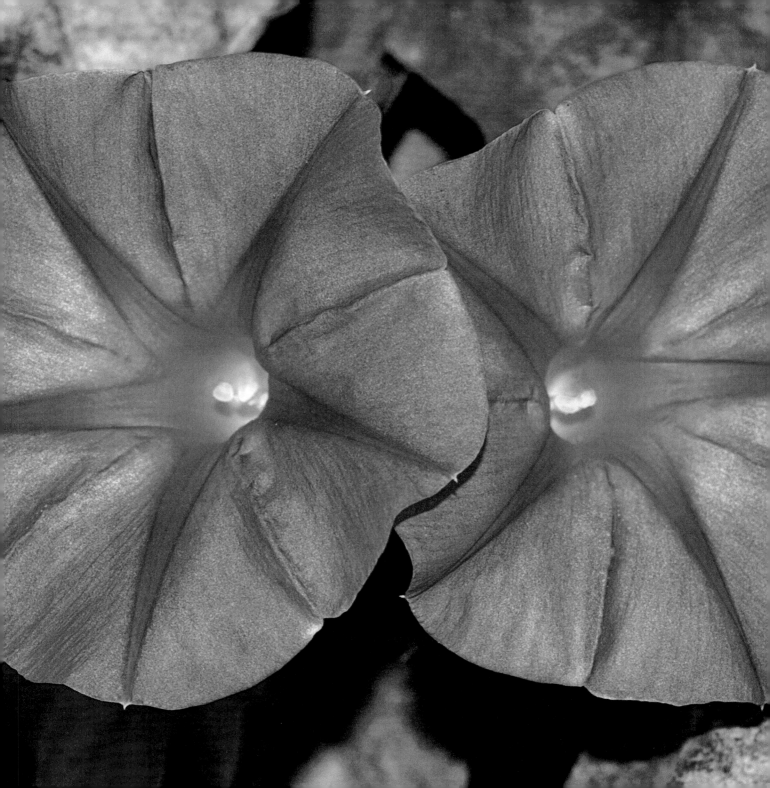

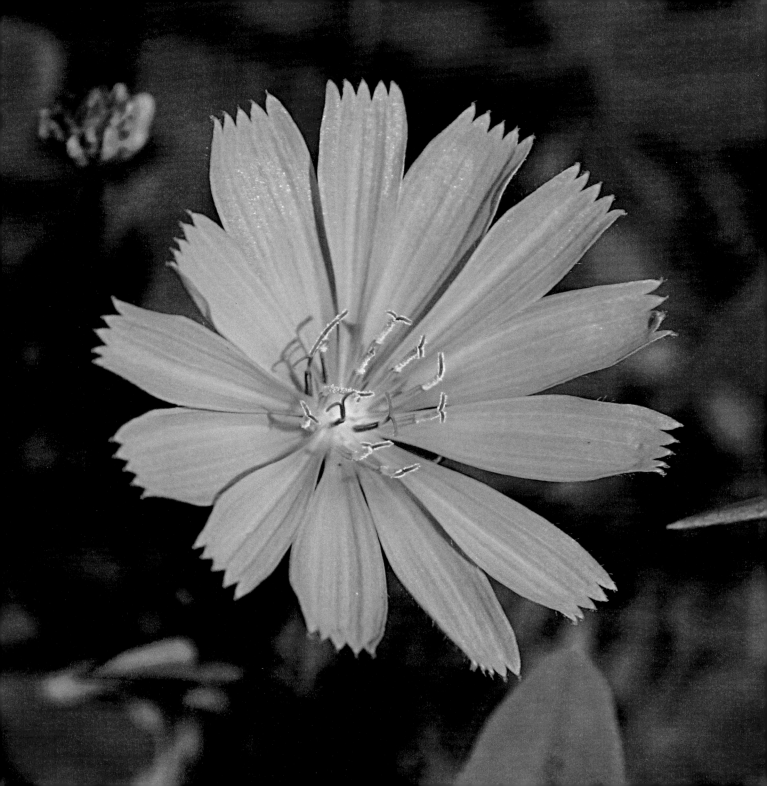

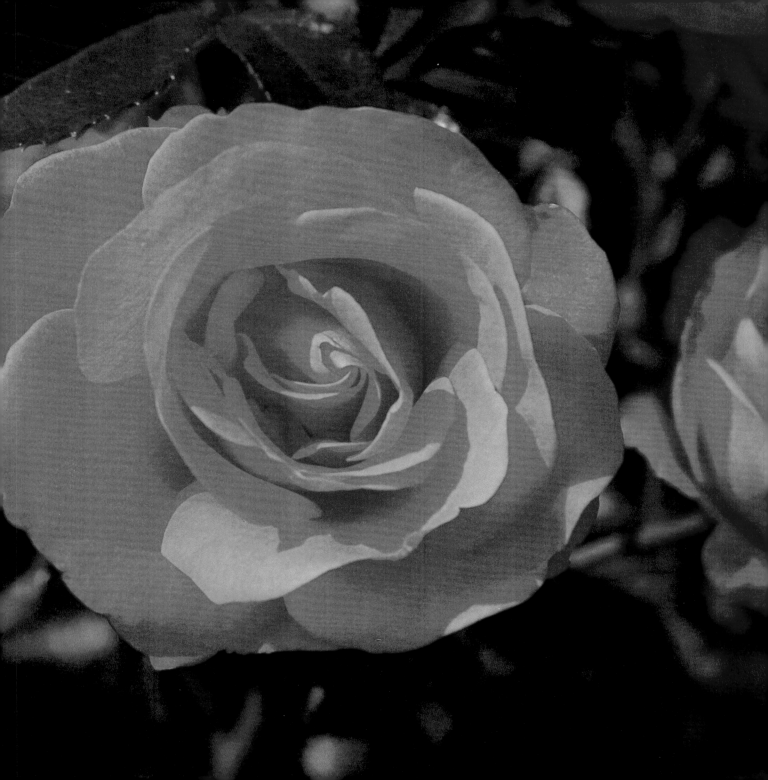

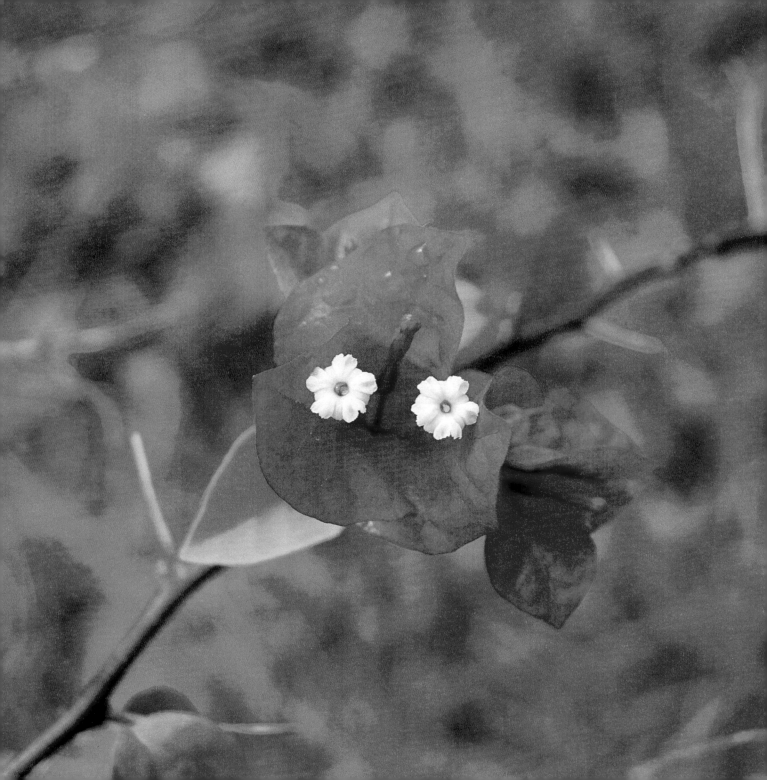

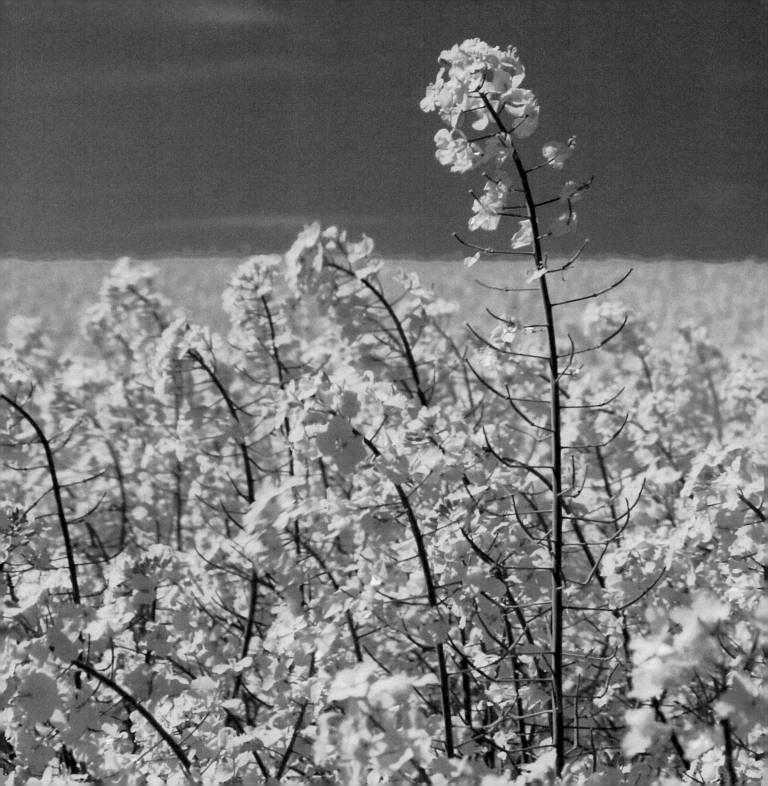

Beautiful-pink-flower - West Virginia - ForestWander
2011-02-12
ForestWander
http://www.forestwander.com/2011/02/beautiful-pink-flower-2/
Creative Commons Attribution-Share Alike 3.0 us

Balsamorhiza sagittata
2009-06-14
Matthew P. Del Buono
Own work
Creative Commons Attribution-Share Alike 3.0

Clematis Etoile Violette
2010-07-08 09:57
johnson from Cotswold Hills, England, England
Clematis "Etoile Violette"

Uploaded by uleli

Creative Commons Attribution 2.0

Cyclamen persicum Mill 08DEC06
2008-12-06
???? (talk)masaki ikeda
SELF made?camera location:My Greenhouse
Public domain

Cynara cardunculus - open - Anstey 2008
2009-01
Peripitus
Own work
Creative Commons Attribution-Share Alike 3.0

Cosmos bipinnatus 06 ies
2007-09-18 12:11:43
Frank Vincentz
Own work
Creative Commons Attribution-Share Alike 3.0

Anthyllis vulneraria, AlpenWundklee 1
2008-07-06
Böhringer
Own work
Creative Commons Attribution-Share Alike 2.5

Dipladenia 2 FR 2013
2013-05-17 15:55:28
JLPC
Own work
Creative Commons Attribution-Share Alike 3.0

Arnica montana
2006-08-03

Calluna vulgaris (15154935468)
2014-09-21 13:47
Joan Simon from Barcelona, España
Calluna vulgaris

Dubium FR 2013
2013-05-17 15:19:19
JLPC
Own work

Carlina corymbosa Corse
2013-08-22
Myrabella
Own work

Digitalis grandiflora-Kaernten-2008-Thomas Huntke
2008-07-13
Thomas Huntke, Germany (der Uploader) http://www.huntke.de
Own work (Original text: Eigenes Foto)

Chrysanthemum coronarium May 2008
2008-05-07
Laitche

Link to My Website.
Own work

Echium auberianum LC0202
2009-06-04
Jörg Hempel
Own work

Geranium pratense (Meadow Cranesbill)
2009-06-14
Julie Anne Workman
Own work

Flowers March 2008-19
2008-04
Alvesgaspar
Own work

Frühlings Enzian Gentiana verna 09

2009-05-19
böhringer friedrich
Own work
Creative Commons Attribution-Share Alike 2.5

Echium April 2010-2
2010-04
Alvesgaspar
Own work
Creative Commons Attribution-Share Alike 3.0

Echinops Ain France
2006-04-23
User:Stephane8888 (Stephane8888 Wiktionnaire)
http://commons.wikimedia.org/wiki/Main Page
Creative Commons Attribution-Share Alike 2.5

Bella Rosa (Kordes 1981)
2008-07-23
Huhu. The original uploader was Huhu at German Wikipedia
selbst fotografiert im Rosarium UetersenTransferred from de.wikipedia to Commons by Anna reg using CommonsHelper.
Public domain

Hydrangea macrophylla 02
2007-06-24
Marc Ryckaert (MJJR)
Own work
Creative Commons Attribution 2.5

Hibiscus petal
2006-01-15
Nvineeth
Own work
Creative Commons Attribution-Share Alike 3.0

Felicia amelloides03
2007-01-04
KENPEI
KENPEI's photo
Creative Commons Attribution-Share Alike 3.0

Daffodil field in Northern Washington
2005-03-28 13:37
Cyprien Lomas
originally posted to Flickr as Northern Washington
Creative Commons Attribution-Share Alike 2.0

Hyacint2

I.Sáček, senior
Own work
Public domain

Flor Maracujá chapada diamantina
2015-05-03 16:56:48
Karina m roque
Own work
Creative Commons Attribution-Share Alike 3.0

Kwiat niebieski 17.08.08 cykoria pl
2008-08-17
Pleple2000
Own work
GNU Free Documentation License

Gentiana asclepiadea 02
2009-08-27
Etienne
Own work
Creative Commons Attribution-Share Alike 3.0

Iris latifolia 01
2010-07-28
Myrabella
Own work
Creative Commons Attribution-Share Alike 3.0

Ipomoea August 2007-1
2007-08
Alvesgaspar
Own work
Creative Commons Attribution 2.5

Encyclia vitellina 1001 Orchids
2013-03-15
Marie-Lan Nguyen
Own work
Creative Commons Attribution 2.5

Erysimum cheiri gold garden flowers
5.13.07
Photo by and (c)2007 Jina Lee
Own work
Creative Commons Attribution-Share Alike 3.0

Globularia punctata (habitus)
2009-05-02
Hans Hillewaert
Own work
Creative Commons Attribution-Share Alike 3.0

Flowers (124)
2007-02-26
Vinayaraj
Own work
Creative Commons Attribution-Share Alike 3.0

93609403R00024

Made in the USA
San Bernardino, CA
09 November 2018